Impact of Sleep Training and Cry it Out

Excerpt from *The Science of Mother-Infant Sleep*

Edited by

**Wendy Middlemiss, PhD and
Kathleen Kendall-Tackett, PhD, IBCLC, FAPA**

Praeclarus Press, LLC

www.PraeclarusPress.com

Praeclarus Press, LLC

2504 Sweetgum Lane

Amarillo, Texas 79124 USA

806-367-9950

www.PraeclarusPress.com

DISCLAIMER

The information contained in this publication is advisory only and is not intended to replace sound clinical judgment or individualized patient care. The author disclaims all warranties, whether expressed or implied, including any warranty as the quality, accuracy, safety, or suitability of this information for any particular purpose.

ISBN 978-1-939807-59-5

Cover Design: Ken Tackett
Acquisition & Development: Kathleen Kendall-Tackett
Copy Editing: Chris Tackett
Layout & Design: Nelly Murariu
Operations: Scott Sherwood

Table of Contents

Chapter 1
Why Cry-It-Out and Sleep-Training
Techniques Are Bad for Babes   5

Chapter 2
Dangers of "Crying It Out":
Damaging Children and Their
Relationships for the Long-term   11

Chapter 3
Why Not "Crying It Out" (Part 1)
The Science that Tells Us that
Responsiveness Is Key   21

Chapter 4
Why Not "Crying It Out" (Part 2)
Can Certain Infant Care Practices
Cause Excessive Stress?   37

Chapter 5
The Ethics of Early Life Care:
the Harms of Sleep Training   49

1

Why Cry-It-Out and Sleep-Training Techniques Are Bad for Babes

Kathleen Kendall-Tackett

In 1998, Dr. Dick Krugman, then Editor-in-Chief of the journal *Child Abuse & Neglect*, asked me to write a review of new studies coming out on the neuropsychology of trauma, with a particular focus on the long-term impact of childhood abuse. I was happy to do it. It was an exciting time in the child maltreatment/trauma field.

With new technology, researchers could finally study living human brains. This technology opened up whole new worlds, and I had a chance to summarize these findings for the major journal in my field (Kendall-Tackett, 2000).

The article took months to write. Since research in this field was so new, many of the findings were contradictory. For example, the physiological footprint of major depression was the exact opposite of the footprint for posttraumatic stress disorder (PTSD). How could that be? It was common for one person to have both.

Researchers eventually developed better models that helped us understand these apparently contradictory findings. But in those first few years, they were hard to understand. One finding, however, was remarkably consistent across studies: chronic stress was bad for the brain.

This was true for adults. And it was especially true for children under the age of 5, whose brains are malleable, and therefore highly vulnerable to stress. As Bruce Perry found, ongoing childhood stress could permanently alter the way children's brains worked.

Robert Sapolsky (1996) authored one of the classic articles on the effects of stress in the journal *Science*: Why stress is bad for the brain. In this article, he described the impact of the stress hormone cortisol on the hippocampus, the section of the brain involved in learning and memory. In *in vitro* studies, dripping cortisol on hippocampal cells made them shrink. In living human beings, those who experienced ongoing chronic stress or depression (which elevated cortisol levels), had smaller hippocampi than those without stress or depression. Dr. Doug Bremner and others have found a similar pattern with combat vets and sexual abuse survivors with PTSD (Bremner, 2006). There were many other studies with similar findings. But the bottom line is this: chronically elevated cortisol levels harm brain cells.

So imagine my shock when I first learned that generally well-meaning parents were deliberately subjecting their babies to routines that chronically elevated their cortisol levels. The parents wanted to train their babies to sleep, or to be independent.

Some of these approaches are worse than others, and the milder forms will probably not cause long-term harm if they occur in the context of overall responsive parenting. I'm sure that parents who tried these approaches thought they were doing the right thing. However, if you understand the physiology, how could chronically raising babies' cortisol levels by not responding to them possibly be the right thing?

Although it has not been specifically studied, it is plausible that sleep training and cry-it-out techniques could also harm breastfeeding. Breastfeeding depends on mothers responding to their babies' cues.

Historically, we have seen the disasterous effects of scheduled feeding on breastfeeding. Sleep training, especially when it involves ignoring infants' cries, could have the same effect. Mothers who are told to ignore their babies' cries in some instances will find it more difficult to be responsive to their infants in other instances. This is a case of culture overriding a mother's hard-wired response to her baby.

Spacing out feedings, or stopping night feedings at some arbitrary age, will have a direct impact on a mother's milk production, possibly opening the door to low milk-supply, decreased weight gain, increased supplementation, and even failure to thrive.

In 2013, there were two widely publicized studies, with wide news coverage, that advocated sleep training and "cry it out" techniques. These approaches are vestiges from Behaviorism, a school of thought that dominated American Psychology from the 1920s to the early 1960s. The idea behind sleep training, etc., is that if you respond to crying you are just "reinforcing" it— meaning that you are increasing the likelihood that it will happen again. As these chapters describe, subsequent anthropological and psychological research has demonstrated the opposite to be true. Babies whose cries are answered in infancy tend to cry less in later infancy and beyond.

In addition, chronic stress in infancy and early childhood has been identified as a major contributor to adult health problems. In 2009, Jack Shonkoff and colleagues published a major review in the *Journal of the American Medical Association* that stated that "adult disease prevention begins with reducing early toxic stress." Considering the state of Americans' health, this is something we should take quite seriously. A recent report from the Institute of Medicine (2013) noted the following:

> For many years, Americans have been dying at younger ages than people in almost all other high-income countries. This disadvantage has been getting worse for three decades, especially among women. Not only are their lives shorter, but Americans also have a longstanding pattern of poorer health that is strikingly consistent and pervasive over the life course.

One way we can improve the health of the next generation is to challenge the hegemony of the cry-it-out advocates. We need to stand by the mothers we serve as they make the decision to defy cultural norms and respond to their babies. The health of the next generation depends on it.

References

Bremner, J.D. (2006). Stress and brain atrophy. *CNS and Neurological Disorders Drug Targets, 5*(5), 503-512.

Institute of Medicine. (2013). *U.S. health in international perspective: Shorter lives, poorer health.* Retrieved from: http://www.iom.edu/~/media/Files/Report%20Files/2013/US-HealthInternational-Perspective/USHealth_Intl_PerspectiveRB.pdf

Kendall-Tackett, K. A. (2000). Physiological correlates of childhood abuse: Chronic hyperarousal in PTSD, depression, and irritable bowel syndrome. *Child Abuse & Neglect, 24,* 799-810.

Sapolsky, R.M. (1996). Why stress is bad for your brain. *Science, 273,* 749-750.

Shonkoff, J. P., Boyce, W. T., & McEwen, B. S. (2009). Neuroscience, molecular biology, and the childhood roots of health disparities: Building a new framework for health promotion and disease prevention. *JAMA, 301*(21), 2252-2259.

Dangers of "Crying It Out": Damaging Children and Their Relationships for the Long-term

Darcia Narvaez

L etting babies "cry it out" is an idea that has been around since at least the 1880s, when the field of medicine was in a hullaballoo about germs and transmitting infection, and so took to the notion that babies should rarely be touched (see Blum, 2002, for a great review of this time period and attitudes towards childrearing).

In the 20th century, behaviorist John Watson (1928), interested in making psychology a hard science, took up the crusade against affection as president of the American Psychological Association. He applied the mechanistic paradigm of Behaviorism to childrearing, warning about the dangers of too much mother love.

The 20th century was the time when "men of science" were assumed to know better than mothers, grandmothers, and families about how to raise a child. Too much kindness to a baby would result in a whiney, dependent, failed human being. Funny how "the experts" got away with this with no evidence to back it up! Instead there is evidence all around (then and now) showing the opposite to be true.

A government pamphlet from the time recommended that "mothering meant holding the baby quietly, in tranquility-inducing positions," and that "the mother should stop immediately if her arms feel tired" because "the baby is never to inconvenience the adult." Babies older than 6 months "should be taught to sit silently in the crib; otherwise, he might need to be constantly watched and entertained by the mother, a serious waste of time." (See Blum, 2002.)

Don't these attitudes sound familiar? A parent reported to me recently that he was encouraged to let his baby cry herself to sleep so he "could get his life back."

With neuroscience, we can confirm what our ancestors took for granted: that letting babies get distressed is a practice that can damage children and their relational capacities in many ways for the long term. We know now that leaving babies to cry is a good way to make a less intelligent and healthy, but more anxious, uncooperative and alienated person, who can pass the same—or worse—traits on to the next generation.

The discredited view sees the baby as an interloper into the life of the parents, an intrusion who must be controlled by various means so the adults can live their lives without too much bother. Perhaps we can excuse this attitude and ignorance because at the time extended families were being broken up, and new parents had to figure out how to deal with babies on their own: an unnatural condition for humanity. We have heretofore raised children in extended families. The parents always shared care with multiple adult relatives.

According to this discredited view, completely ignorant of human development, the child "has to be taught to be independent." We can confirm now that forcing "independence" on a baby leads to greater dependence. Instead, giving babies what they need leads to greater independence later.

In anthropological reports of small-band hunter-gatherers, parents took care of every need of babies and young children. Toddlers felt confident enough (and so did their parents) to walk into the bush on their own (see *Hunter-Gatherer Childhoods*, edited by Hewlett & Lamb, 2005).

Ignorant advisors then—and now—encourage parents to condition the baby to expect needs NOT to be met on demand, whether feeding or comforting. It's assumed that the adults should "be in charge" of the relationship. Certainly this might foster a child that doesn't ask for as much help and attention (withdrawing into depression and going into stasis—or even wasting away), but it is more likely to foster a whiny, unhappy, aggressive, and/or demanding child: one who has learned that one must scream to get needs met. A deep sense of insecurity is likely to stay with them for the rest of their lives.

The fact is that caregivers who habitually respond to the needs of the baby before the baby gets distressed, preventing crying, are more likely to have children who are independent than the opposite (e.g., Stein & Newcomb, 1994). Soothing care is best from the outset. Once patterns get established, it's much harder to change them.

We should understand the mother and child as a mutually responsive dyad. They are a symbiotic unit that make each other healthier and happier in mutual responsiveness. This expands to other caregivers too.

One strangely popular notion still around today is to let babies "cry it out" when they are left alone, isolated in cribs or other devices. This comes from a misunderstanding of child and brain development.

1. Babies grow from being held. Their bodies get dysregulated when they are physically separated from caregivers.

2. Babies indicate a need through gesture and eventually, if necessary, through crying. Just as adults reach for liquid when thirsty, children search for what they need in the moment. Just as adults become calm once the need is met, so do babies.

3. There are many long-term effects of under care, or need-neglect, in babies (e.g., Dawson et al., 2000).

What does "crying it out" actually do to the baby and to the dyad?

Neurons Die

When the baby is stressed, the toxic hormone cortisol is released. It's a neuron killer. A full-term baby (40 to 42 weeks), with only 25% of its brain developed, is undergoing rapid brain growth. The brain grows, on average, three times as large by the end of the first year (and head size growth in the first year is a sign of intelligence, e.g., Gale et al., 2006).

Who knows what neurons are not being connected, or being wiped out during times of extreme stress? What deficits might show up years later from such regular distressful experience?

Disordered stress reactivity can be established as a pattern for life not only in the brain with the stress-response system, but also in the body through the vagus nerve, a nerve that affects functioning in multiple systems (e.g., digestion). For example, prolonged distress in early life, resulting in a poorly functioning vagus nerve, is related to disorders, such as irritable bowel syndrome (Stam et al., 1997). (See more about how early stress is toxic for lifelong health from the recent Harvard report, *The Foundations of Lifelong Health are Built in Early Childhood*).

Self-regulation is Undermined

The baby is absolutely dependent on caregivers for learning how to self-regulate. Responsive care—meeting the baby's needs before he gets distressed—tunes the body and brain up for calmness. When a baby gets scared, and a parent holds and comforts him, the baby builds expectations for soothing, which get integrated into the ability to self-comfort.

Babies don't self-comfort in isolation. If they are left to cry alone, they learn to shut down in face of extensive distress—stop growing, stop feeling, stop trusting (Henry & Wang, 1998).

Trust is Undermined

As Erik Erikson pointed out, the first year of life is a sensitive period for establishing a sense of trust in the world, the world of caregiver, and the world of self. When a baby's needs are met without distress, the child learns that the world is a trustworthy place, that relationships are supportive, and that the self is a positive entity that can get its needs met.

When a baby's needs are dismissed or ignored, the child develops a sense of mistrust of relationships and the world. And self-confidence is undermined. The child may spend a lifetime trying to fill the inner emptiness.

Caregiver responsiveness to the needs of the baby is related to most—if not all—positive child outcomes

In our work, caregiver responsiveness is related to intelligence, empathy, lack of aggression or depression, self-regulation, and social competence. Because responsiveness is so powerful, we have to control for it in our studies of other parenting practices and child outcomes.

The importance of caregiver responsiveness is common knowledge in developmental psychology. Lack of responsiveness, which "crying it out" represents, can result in the opposite of the aforementioned positive outcomes.

The "cry it out" approach seems to have arisen as a solution to the dissolution of extended family life in the 20th century. The vast wisdom of grandmothers was lost in the distance between households with children, and those with the experience and expertise about how to raise them well. The wisdom of keeping babies happy was lost between generations.

But isn't it normal for babies to cry?

No. A crying baby in our ancestral environment would have signaled predators to tasty morsels. So our evolved parenting practices alleviated baby distress and precluded crying except in emergencies. Babies are built to expect the equivalent of an "external womb" after birth (see Allan Schore, specific references below). What is the external womb?—being held constantly, breastfed on demand, and needs met quickly.

These practices are known to facilitate good brain and body development. When babies display discomfort, it signals that a need is not getting met, a need of their rapidly growing systems.

What does extensive baby crying signal?

It shows the lack of experience, knowledge, and/or support of the baby's caregivers. To remedy a lack of information in us all, I listed a good set of articles about all the things that a baby's cry can signal. We can all educate ourselves about what babies need and the practices that alleviate baby crying. We can help one another to keep it from happening as much as possible.

For Further Reading

Blum, D. (2002). *Love at Goon Park: Harry Harlow and the science of affection*. New York: Berkeley Publishing (Penguin).

Dawson, G., et al. (2000). The role of early experience in shaping behavioral and brain development and its implications for social policy. *Development and Psychopathology, 12*(4), 695-712.

Gale, C.R., O'Callaghan, F.J., Bredow, M., Martyn, C.N., and the Avon Longitudinal Study of Parents and Children Study Team. (2006). The influence of head growth in fetal life, infancy, and childhood on intelligence at the ages of 4 and 8 years. *Pediatrics, 118*(4), 1486-1492.

Henry, J.P., & Wang, S. (1998). Effects of early stress on adult affiliative behavior. *Psychoneuroendocrinology, 23*(8), 863-875.

Hewlett, B., & Lamb, M. (2005). *Hunter-gatherer childhoods*. New York: Aldine.

Meaney, M.J. (2001). Maternal care, gene expression, and the transmission of individual differences in stress reactivity across generations. *Annual Review of Neuroscience, 24,* 1161-1192.

Narvaez, D., Panksepp, J., Schore, A., & Gleason, T. (Eds.) (2013). *Evolution, early experience and human development: From research to practice and policy.* New York: Oxford University Press.

Schore, A.N. (1997). Early organization of the nonlinear right brain and development of a predisposition to psychiatric disorders. *Development and Psychopathology, 9,* 595-631.

Schore, A.N. (2000). Attachment and the regulation of the right brain. *Attachment & Human Development, 2,* 23-47.

Schore, A.N. (2001). The effects of early relational trauma on right brain development, affect regulation, and infant mental health. *Infant Mental Health Journal, 22,* 201-269.

Stein, J. A., & Newcomb, M. D. (1994). Children's internalizing and externalizing behaviors and maternal health problems. *Journal of Pediatric Psychology, 19*(5), 571-593.

UNICEF (2007). *Child poverty in perspective: An overview of child well-being in rich countries, a comprehensive assessment of the lives and well-being of children and adolescents in the economically advanced nations,* Report Card 7. Florence, Italy: United Nations Children's Fund Innocenti Research Centre.

U.S. Department of Health and Human Services, Substance Abuse and Mental Health Services Administration. (1999). *Mental health: A report of the Surgeon General.* Rockville, MD: Center for Mental Health Services, National Institutes of Health, National Institute of Mental Health.

Watson, J. B. (1928). *Psychological care of infant and child.* New York: W. W. Norton Company.

WHO/WONCA (2008). *Integrating mental health into primary care: A global perspective.* Geneva and London: World Health Organization and World Organization of Family Doctors.

3

Why Not "Crying It Out" (Part 1)
The Science that Tells Us that Responsiveness Is Key

Patrice Marie Miller
Michael Lamport Commons

Considerable research, both experimental research with animals and research with humans, now documents the detrimental effects of early stress on brain development. These effects can occur not just in response to intense and repetitive stressful situations, but with some probability may also occur in situations of parenting that is not responsive. In this context, this chapter addresses the biologically and ethologically based reasons that crying is detrimental to infants' development—negatively impacting neurological structures, stress responses, physical health, and socioemotional well-being.

From birth, human infants have a limited ability to control their environment. If distressed, they will usually cry, but it is not up to them what happens in response to that cry. Infants have limited self-soothing abilities (Emde, 1998), and are reliant upon an appropriate response from caregivers. Of course, as they develop, their response repertoires increase so that they may be responded to more effectively, and their own coping and self-soothing behaviors also develop.

It remains true, however, that the successful development of an infant, and even a young child, is due to an intricate, interactive process between that child and its caregivers. In that context, the number and kinds of stressful events (or "stressors") that an infant encounters in the course of a day is a factor that may have a major effect on their development.

While caregivers cannot totally eliminate stressors, they can have major control over the number and kinds of stressful events. Caregivers can impact infants' experiences of stressors as well by being present, holding, and/or otherwise consoling an infant during a stressful event.

The purpose of this chapter is to examine a large body of evidence on the effect of early stressors on development. In "Why Not 'Crying It Out,' Part 2," we examine common care practices in some cultures, such as northern Euro-American cultures, that can produce excessive stress for some infants and young children. What mitigates against these stressors is re-adopting practices familiar to professionals and protective of infants' development.

These practices can include co-sleeping or parent-settling sleep, increasing the rate of bodily contact and holding, and other responsive care behaviors. The argument for these mitigating practices will be presented based on this evidence.

Evidence for the Negative Effects of Stress on Development

The literature on the effects of early stressful events on development has been growing by leaps and bounds for roughly the last 15 years. The evidence for these effects comes from two sources: (a) experimental research on animals, such as rats or monkeys, which combines controlled exposure to stressful events with examination of brain changes and behavior, and (b) research involving human children and adults that relates different kinds of early experiences to brain changes and/or to behavior in a correlational fashion. Each will be briefly reviewed in turn.

Effects of Stressful Events on Brain Development in Non-Human Animals

Recognizing that we are mammals is an important step in helping to understand the importance of early care. Because of the nature of development, researchers and scientists are able to explore the connection between care and brain development—particularly with regard to early care and the impact on later behavior—more readily than they might if working with new parents and infants.

The information gathered has provided substantial support that solidifies the importance of early care. The strength of this support is presented here as a means of assuring professionals of the value and importance of the sleep and care routines often recommended.

Biological Importance of Maternal Care

A number of investigators have studied the long-term effects of stressful early rearing conditions in non-human animals. Some of the early research in this area provides a clear look into the importance of care in shaping later behavior. In their research using rhesus monkeys, Suomi and colleagues (1987; 1991) have investigated the differential effects of being reared by their mother in the traditional way, or by being separated from the mother and being reared by peers.

Peer-reared monkeys seemed to develop relatively normal social behavior as long as they were in familiar settings. When exposed to stressors, such as separations from other monkeys, however, they exhibited much more behavioral disruption, and a greater activation of the hypothalamic-pituitary-adrenal axis and other systems involved in dealing with stress.

Suomi (1987) also reported that there were important individual differences in the reactivity of different individual monkeys, with roughly 20% of them being highly reactive to stress. Even when mother-reared, these monkeys showed much more extreme behavioral and physiological reactions to stressful situations. They might, for example, appear fearful in novel situations and have heightened levels of cortisol and ACTH (adrenocorticotropic hormone).

These patterns of behavior, both from monkeys who were reared by peers, and in the highly reactive monkeys, have been found to persist into later development.

Stressful Environments and Caregiving

Research continues to support these earlier findings. In an extensive review of studies with rodents and also non-human primates, Sánchez, Ladd, and Plotsky (2001) summarized a great deal of evidence showing the role of stress in early rearing for both rodents and primates. What was evident through the review was that early adverse experiences, including prenatal stress or illness in the mother and separations from the mother, for either brief or extended periods of time, changes the way that the limbic-hypothalamic-pituitary-adrenal (LHPA) axis is regulated.

While the negative effects on this stress-regulation system have been shown to vary somewhat in different individuals and during different periods of development, across all the species studied, a number of similar effects were seen. These included: "increase in fearfulness and anxiety-like behavior, and...deficits in social behavior, sexual behavior, and cognitive performance" (p. 440, Sánchez et al.).

One interesting finding that is also part of this literature is that for rodents, certain caregiving behaviors from the mother, specifically licking and grooming of the pups during the first 10 days, led to reduced levels of plasma adrenocorticotropic hormone, as well as other responses to stress (Liu et al., 1997). According to the authors, an important function of maternal behavior is to "program" the regulation of the LHPA axis. We will argue (below) that the same is true in humans.

Research on Effects of Stressful Events on Human Behavior and Brain Development

The long-term effects of early stress experiences have been found to be much the same in humans. Sources of stress examined in regard to infants' well-being have included studies regarding trauma or abuse in infancy (e.g., Essex, Klein, Cho & Kalin, 2002; Ito, Teicher, Glod, & Ackerman, 1998; Perry, 1997).

Other literature discusses stressors that a significant number of children are exposed to, including low socioeconomic status (Lupien et al., 2000), stress due to maternal depression (e.g., Ashman et al., 2002; Essex et al., 2002), and simply "low-quality maternal behavior" (Hane & Fox, 2006). This body of research has been summarized both by the National Scientific Council on the Development of the Child (2005), and Shonkoff and colleagues (2012).

These latter reports, in particular, include evidence showing that there are short- and long-term effects on both mental and physical health when children grow up in stressful environments. Exposure to chronic stress seems to be associated with physical disorders (for example, cardiovascular disease, cancer), and also psychological disorders, such as depression and anxiety (see McEwen & Seeman, 1999).

In some studies, exposure to high amounts of cortisol that is released in response to stressors has been shown to result in damage to the hippocampus (involved in learning and memory; e.g., Lupien et al., 1998), and the amygdala (involved in the processing of emotions; e.g., Wolterink et al., 2001).

Why This Is Important

During the first years of life, a child's experiences of stress will begin to shape the functioning of their stress-response systems. When infancy is marked by acute or chronic stress experiences, the impact on this system can be irreversible, leading to the development of an overactive, intense response system to stress, or a dampening of response (Gunnar, 1998).

Infants' first experiences are crucial for the developing hypothalamic-pituitary-adrenocortical (HPA) axis because this system is very responsive to stimulation. This can be seen by parents and care providers in infants' experiences of everyday events, even minor events, such as being undressed. In her work, Gunnar has found that infants can experience elevations in cortisol during these caretaking activities (Gunnar,

1992). Some infants may be more sensitive to these events based on being temperamentally more reactive. The findings of this kind of research are very much echoed in the findings from the research reported by Sánchez, Ladd, and Plotsky (2001), among many others.

The sum of this research, conducted across different populations and using many different methodologies, suggests that exposure to stressors early in life can rearrange certain systems in the brain, particularly the limbic-hypothalamic-pituitary-adrenal (LHPA) axis, which responds to stress.

Dysregulation of the LHPA axis is related to both physiological changes that are related to physical illnesses, and to psychopathology (see Caldji et al., 2001; DeBellis et al., 1994; Heims, Owens, Plotsky, & Nemeroff, 1997; Young, Abelson, Curtis, & Nesse, 1997). Most importantly, these effects appear to be present along a continuum of stressor severity, from severe stressors, such as separations from the mother, to those that are less severe.

What Kind of Model Should We Use When Thinking about the Effects of Stress?

In thinking about the possible effects of stressful events, it is important for parents, and those working directly with parents, to have an explanatory model that fits the results that are described. With such a model, it would be possible to address some of the typical early care questions parents may raise.

Questions might include whether an equally severe form of stress could be expected to have the same kinds of effects on all individuals? Are these characteristics of individuals, or are there other events that might mitigate these possible effects?

A Model Helpful for Working with Families

Currently, one can best describe the explanatory models of the field as consisting of multilevel-dynamic systems accounts, in which characteristics of individuals, as well as contexts, are both important in understanding outcomes of development.

According to Sameroff (2010), the self consists of interacting psychological and biological processes, resulting in a biopsychological self-system. In this system, psychological processes include social behaviors, cognitive and emotional intelligence, and mental health, while the biological processes include the nervous system and neuroendocrine systems among other processes.

The system then interacts within the settings of family, school, etc. This transactional model of development suggests a system of back and forth influences between the biology of the individual, and the characteristics of the various environments that the individual interacts within. That is, a biological change may affect an individual's behavior, which might then elicit changes in the environment. That changed environment can then impinge on the biological systems that started the cycle in the first place.

These transactions have to be considered over time, and in the context of how the individual is changing. In general, in examining the influence of negative events, such as stress, research has relied on what is called the diathesis-stress model (e.g., see paper by Caspi and co-authors, 2002), in which a biological vulnerability of some kind is shown to worsen the effects of stress.

Model Application

This model helps to explain what professionals know from working with families. However, in this application, the professional now has the tools and explanations to help mothers understand the importance of seeing their infants as individuals, and their relationship with the infants as impacting their system of interaction.

A second new development in the field helps to make even more clear the importance of the interaction between mothers and infants—a relationship that the professional has the capacity to discuss with mothers. This development is the recognition of a more general "differential susceptibility" to experiences (Belsky, 1997). For example, in studies of the effects of children's early experiences in child care, few overall negative effects of child care were found.

When researchers focused only on children with negative temperaments, however, they found that these children were both more negatively affected by low-quality care environments, and more positively affected by high-quality care environments (Pluess & Belsky, 2009).

Keeping these models in mind will be useful when considering whether some infant care practices, that are used by many parents in this and other cultures, could cause significant enough stress to change an infant's developmental course to one that is less than optimal.

References

Ashman, S. B. Dawson, G., Panagiotides, H., Yamada, E. & Wilkinson, C. W. (2002). *Development and Psychopathology, 14*(2), 333-349.

Belsky, J. (1997). Variation in susceptibility to rearing influences: An evolutionary argument. *Psychological Inquiry,* 8, 182–186.

Caldji, C., Liu, D., Sharma, S., Diorio, J., Francis, D., Meaney, M., & Plotsky, P. M. (2001). Development of individual differences in behavioral and endocrine responses to stress: Role of the postnatal environment. In B. S. Ewen (Ed.), *Handbook of physiology: Coping with the environment* (pp. 271-292). New York: Oxford University Press.

DeBellis, M. D., Chrousos, G. P., Dom, L. D., Burke, L., Helmers, K., Kling, M.A., Trickett, P.K., & Putnam, F. W. (1994). Hypothalamic pituitary adrenal dysregulation in sexually abused girls. *Journal of Clinical Endocrinology and Metabolism, 78*, 249-255.

Emde, R. N. (1998). Early emotional development: New modes of thinking for research and intervention. In J. G. Warhol & S. P. Shelov (Eds.), *New perspectives in early emotional development.* Johnson & Johnson Pediatric Institute, Ltd.

Essex, M. J., Klein, M. H., Cho, E., & Kalin, N. H. (2002). Maternal stress beginning in infancy may sensitize children to later stress exposure: Effects on cortisol and behavior. *Biological Psychiatry, 52,* 776-784.

Gunnar, M. R. (1992). Reactivity of the hypothalamic-pituitary-adrenocortical system to stressors in normal infants and children. *Pediatrics (Suppl), 90*(3), 491-497.

Gunnar, M. R. (1998). Quality of early care and buffering of neuroendocrine stress reactions: Potential effects on the developing human brain. *Preventive Medicine, 27*, 208-211.

Hane, A. A., & Fox, N. A. (2006). Ordinary variations in maternal caregiving influence human infants' stress reactivity. *Psychological Science, 17*(6), 550-556.

Heim, C., Owens, M. J., Plotsky, P. M., & Nemeroff, C. B. (1997). The role of early adverse life events in the etiology of depression and posttraumatic stress disorder: Focus on corticotropin-releasing factor. *Annals of the New York Academy of Sciences USA, 821,* 194-207.

Ito, Y., Teicher, M. H., Glod, C. A., & Ackerman, E. (1998). Preliminary evidence for aberrant cortical development in abused children: A quantitative EEG study. *Journal of Neuropsychiatry and Clinical Neurosciences, 10,* 298-307.

Liu, D., Diorio, J., Tannenbaum, B., Caldji, C., Francis, D., Freedman, A., Sharma, S., Pearson, D., Plotsky, P. M., & Meaney, M. J. (1997). Maternal care, hippocampal glucocorticoid receptors, and hypothalamic-pituitary-adrenal responses to stress. *Science, 277* (Issue 5332), 1659-1663.

Luecken, L. J. (1998). Childhood attachment and low experiences affect adult cardiovascular and cortisol function. *Psychosomatic Medicine, 60,* 765-772.

Lupien, S. J., King, S., Meaney, M. J., & McEwen, B. S. (2001). Can poverty get under your skin? Basal cortisol levels and cognitive function in children from low and high socioeconomic status. *Developmental Psychopathology, 13,* 653–676.

McEwen, B. S., & Seeman, T. (1999). Protective and damaging effects of mediators of stress: Elaborating and testing the concepts of allostatis and allostatic load. In N. E. Adler, M. Marmot, B. S. McEwen, & J. Steward (Eds.), Socioeconomic status and health in industrial nations: Social, psychological and biological pathways. *Annals of the New York Academy of Sciences, 896,* 30-47.

National Council on the Developing Child (2005). *Excessive stress disrupts the architecture of the developing brain.* Working paper No. 3. Retrieved from: http://www.developingchild.net/reports.shtml.

Perry, B. D. (1997). Incubated in terror: Neurodevelopmental factors in the "Cycle of Violence." In J. Osofsky (Ed.), *Children, youth and violence: The search for solutions* (pp. 124-148). New York: Guilford.

Pluess, M., & Belsky, J. (2009). Differential susceptibility to rearing experience: The case of childcare. *Journal of Child Psychology and Psychiatry and Allied Disciplines, 50*(4), 396–404.

Rosenblum, L. A., Coplan, J. D., Friedman, S., Bassoff, T., Gorman, J. M., & Andrews, M. W. (1994). Adverse early experiences affect noradrenergic and serotonergic functioning in adult primates. *Biological Psychiatry, 35,* 221-227.

Sameroff, A. (2010). A unified theory of development: A dialectic integration of nature and nurture. *Child Development, 81,* 6-22.

Sánchez, M. M., Ladd, C. O., & Plotsky, P.M. (2001). Early adverse experience as a developmental risk factor for later psychopathology: Evidence from rodent and primate models. *Development and Psychopathology, 13,* 419-449.

Shonkoff, J. P., & Garner, A.S., The Committee on Psychosocial Aspects of Child and Family Health, Committee on Early Childhood, Adoption and Dependent Care, and Section on Developmental and Behavioral Pediatrics, Siegel, B. S., Dobbins, M. I, Earls, M. F., McGuinn, L., Pascoe, J., & Wood, D. L. (2012). The lifelong effects of early childhood adversity and toxic stress. *Pediatrics, 129*(1), 232-246.

Suomi, S. J. (1987). Genetic and environmental contributions to individual differences in rhesus monkey biobehavioral development. In N. Krasnegor, E. Blass, M. Hofer, and W. Smotherman (Eds.), *Perinatal development: A psychobiological perspective* (pp. 397-420). New York: Academic Press.

Suomi, A. J. (1991). Early stress and adult emotional reactivity in rhesus monkeys. In G. R. Bock & J. Whelan (Eds.), *CIBA Foundation Symposium: Childhood environment and adult disease.* New York: Wiley.

Wolterink, G., Lisette, E. W., Daenen, P. M., Dubbeldam, S., Mirgam, A. F., Gerrits, M., van Rijn, R., Cruse, C. G., Van Der Haijden, J. A. M., & Van Ree, J. M. (2001).

Early amygdala damage in the rat as a model for neurodevelopmental psychopathological disorders. *European Neuropsychopharamacology, 11*(1), 51-59.

Young, E. A., Abelson, J. L., Curtis, C. G., & Nesse, R. M. (1997). Childhood adversity and vulnerability to mood and anxiety disorders. *Depression Anxiety, 5,* 66-72.

4

Why Not "Crying It Out" (Part 2)
Can Certain Infant Care Practices Cause Excessive Stress?

Patrice Marie Miller
Michael Lamport Commons

Understanding the importance of responsiveness is an essential foundation for communicating with parents about early care. Helping parents create healthy, responsive environments may benefit from looking at some common parenting practices and how they may impact infants' development. The role of stress experiences is an essential consideration when choosing care. What practices may be more risky for infants and which may be more protective is the focus of Part 2.

In Part 1 of "Why Not Crying It Out," we reviewed the science forming the foundation for the importance of communicating to mothers about how they provide early care. This science helps to show how early care will impact infants' developing brains and stress responses, how this aspect of neurological development will impact later behavior.

The next important question to be answered for professionals, and then shared with parents, is whether there are some relatively routine practices used by parents in the United States (and some other countries) that may be stressful enough to affect infants' development. Based on the science then—the question is whether these practices could produce changes in infants' brains and behaviors in the ways indicated by the research on stress and its effects.

Explored here are practices often associated with crying it out—practices such as putting infants to bed by themselves, and allowing them to cry instead of picking them up when they do not fall asleep; or allowing infants to cry and not picking them up when they wake up at night.

Other similar practices marked by parents' non-response would include showing a relative lack of response to crying during the day time (so as not to "spoil" the baby), not holding or touching the baby very much, and so on. We will explore these practices from the framework of parent- and child-centered practices (Miller & Commons, 2010), tying these different practices back to the research reviewed above, and examining the impact of these practices on children's development.

Parent-Centered Versus Child-Centered Parenting with Infants

Child-Centered Practices and Infant Sleep

Child-centered parenting involves learning to read the cues of the infant, and responding appropriately to those cues. Thus, child-centered parenting practices can encompass a variety of parenting strategies, such as feeding in a manner that is responsive to infant cues, and being highly responsive to crying, or pre-crying, as well as to other cues, co-sleeping or responding to infants during nighttime care, and emphasizing bodily contact more than physical separation. A main result of such practices is a reduction in stressful situations for the infant.

In regard to sleeping patterns, practices in which parents attend to infant signaling can provide a child-centered focus. Additionally, co-sleeping can be viewed as child-centered as this nighttime care practice allows for much faster responsiveness to infant cues. With this practice, infants who co-sleep will not be exposed to the extended crying that can occur when they are left alone to fall asleep on their own, or when their parents do not retrieve them from their crib at night.

Having infants co-sleep or sleep in close proximity to parents, rather than in a physically separate crib or a crib in a separate room, can greatly mitigate or completely eliminate problems that a parent may have in getting their infant to sleep, and in dealing with night wakefulness (Miller & Commons, 2010). In addition, mother-infant sleep positions can lead to safer sleep (McKenna & McDade, 2005), as well as enhance the quality of sleep (Teti, Kim, Mayer, & Countermine, 2010), and offer a greater probability of continued breastfeeding (McKenna & McDade, 2005).

Child-Centered Practices and Infants' Crying

One important area of behavior to examine is how quickly and how often mothers and other caregivers respond to infant crying. Infants who are less often responded to, or who are not responded to very quickly, are likely to experience more stress.

This topic overlaps somewhat with the topic of infant holding, since picking up and holding would be a frequent response to crying, along with other behaviors. The distinction is that here, what is being looked at is the presence of a contingent response. The research on responsiveness to crying has not looked at the specific nature of responses to crying, only at how often parents (usually mothers) respond.

This topic was discussed in some detail in Miller and Commons (2010), so here we will present just a summary. Two opposing points of view have been put forward. One, more on the child-centered side, has suggested that responding to infant crying in a timely and contingent fashion reduces the rate of such crying (Bell & Ainsworth, 1972).

The other side suggests that responding to infant crying could actually increase the rate of infant crying, because the rate of crying essentially becomes strengthened or reinforced when responded to (Gewirtz & Boyd, 1977). This overall controversy seems central to the discussion about whether infants should be left to "cry it out" at any time.

In one study, St. James-Roberts et al. (2006) compared parents who held their infants a great deal of the time (on average 15 to 16 hours per day) versus those who held them much less. They found that the infants who were held much less cried 50% more overall.

Clearly the holding of infants is another important behavior that can reduce how stressed infants and their caregivers might be. This is supported by studies that show that infant crying is an important cause or at least precipitating event for abuse and maltreatment in a number of cases (Soltis, 2004).

Other Positive Socialization Benefits of Child-Centered Parenting

One of the additional benefits of child-centered parenting could be a closer sense of "connection" to other people. Because physical contact and touching is a less salient aspect of Western, and particularly Northern European cultures, this possible benefit has rarely been studied.

At the very least, parents who engage in highly responsive caregiving serve as models for their children. Thereby, they may promote higher frequencies of responsive, and even empathetic behavior toward others, as also noted by Bandura (1989).

Discussion and Conclusions

We have presented evidence that a number of child-centered practices may promote optimal development in a variety of ways. The discussion has focused primarily on practices that are related to soothing infants and reducing arousal, as these are most important, particularly during the early months, as far as buffering the infant against stressful events.

We have argued that reducing the number and kinds of early stressful events are important, having possible consequences both for the development of children's brains, and for their behavior. The argument is, that as seen in rodents and other mammals, the caregiver plays an important role, through his or her practices, in helping to tune or program the infant's stress-regulation system.

As infants continue to develop in many ways including attachment (Commons, 1991), their behavior and physiology changes. We have argued that the need for child-centered parenting does not end after the first few months of life, but that it continues, accommodating itself to developmental changes in young children (Miller & Commons, 2010).

To give one example, as children become more mobile, they will spend more time away from their parents and not being held. As research has also shown (e.g., Anderson, 1972), when the child initiates the departure from contact, and can rely on the parent remaining in the same location, they are more likely to freely explore.

When the parent initiates the separation, children have a great deal more trouble coping. In this case, children will be more likely to protest, and if possible to return to the parent's side (e.g., Ainsworth et al., 1978). Miller and Commons (2010) discuss several other possible changes in parenting behavior that might take place.

Parenting Behaviors that Cause Infant Stress Are Normative in the U.S.

It has to be noted that the types of parenting behaviors that might cause stress are considered by a large part of the population in the United States to be normative. As discussed by LeVine and colleagues (1994), by Richman, Miller, and Solomon (1988) and others, and these behaviors form part of a parenting strategy that emphasizes the infant and child's development of independence from the parent(s).

Parents who use these practices sincerely believe that it is most important to insist that the child behave independently, and that to "give in" to behaviors, such as crying or requests for attention, will simply encourage the child to become dependent. This belief is pervasive in this culture, so parents using "independence-promoting" strategies are, to a large extent, engaging in parenting that fits with the norms.

Individual Differences in Infants' Ability to Tolerate These Practices

Plus it would seem that some infants, and perhaps most, are able to tolerate these practices to some extent. So, some proportion of infants will learn—sooner or later—to fall asleep on their own. Many infants will eventually learn some self-consoling behaviors. As already noted, even though such infants may appear at that time to have mastered these tasks, one sometimes sees that the adaptation is not complete. For example, infants who have been sleeping alone often turn into toddlers and older children who seek comfort in their parents' bed when they are fearful or distressed.

We have also presented studies suggesting that the number of children using self-comfort objects, such as pacifiers, security blankets, or stuffed animals is much larger in the U.S. than in cultures in which infants and children neither sleep by themselves nor are encouraged to self-console (Miller & Commons, 2010).

Secondly, and as noted earlier, there are individual differences in how different infants may respond to the same kind of parenting practices, with some infants being more vulnerable than others. Some infants may seek physical contact more than others, and may not be at all easily consoled without it (Miller & Commons, 2010).

Some infants may be more easily consoled than others. Some infants may continue to sleep best with a parent or parents, whereas others may sleep well separately. The research on differential susceptibility that was cited earlier (Pluess & Belsky, 2009), as well as other studies (e.g., Caspi et al., 2002) have in fact confirmed that a "one size fits all" strategy will not work for every individual.

What Do Infants Learn from Independence-Promoting Strategies?

Even if an infant or child has largely coped with an independence-promoting strategy as opposed to one that is child-centered, as a culture we have to ask ourselves, what have they learned? Ultimately, they have learned that they are essentially alone. The lesson is repeatedly reinforced. If you are distressed, you must deal with it yourself. If you are frightened, don't bother us. The message is that there is "something wrong with you" if you are suffering too much.

Ultimately, this seems designed to not only reduce one's reliance on others, but can have the unintended consequence of our becoming completely alienated from those others. When we have what seems like an ever increasing incidence of lone and very lonely people perpetrating acts of violence against others, it might be that we should, as a culture, start asking the question as to whether the costs of our preferred childrearing strategies might be too high.

References

Ainsworth, M. D. S., Blehar, M. C., Waters, E., & Wall, S. (1978). *Patterns of attachment: A psychological study of the strange situation*. Hillsdale, N.J.: Erlbaum.

Anderson, J. W. (1972). Attachment behavior out of doors. In N. Blurton Jones (Ed.), *Ethological studies of child behavior* (pp. 199-215). Cambridge, U.K.: Cambridge University Press.

Bandura, A. (1989). Social cognitive theory. In R. Vasta (Ed.), *Annals of child development* (Vol. 6, pp. 1-60). Greenwich, CT: JAI Press.

Bell, S. M., & Ainsworth, M.D.S. (1972). Infant crying and maternal responsiveness. *Child Development, 43*, 1171-1190.

Caspi, A., McClay, J., Moffitt, T. E., Mill, J., Judy Martin, J., Craig, I. W., Taylor, A., & Poulton, R. (2002). Role of genotype in the cycle of violence in maltreated children. *Science, 297*(5582), 851-854.

Commons, M. L. (1991). A comparison and synthesis of Kohlberg's Cognitive-Developmental and Gewirtz's Learning-Developmental Attachment Theories. In J. L. Gewirtz & W. M. Kurtines (Eds.), *Intersections with attachment* (pp. 257-291). Hillsdale, NJ: Erlbaum.

Gewirtz, J. L., & Boyd, E. F. (1977). Does maternal responding imply reduced infant crying? A critique of the 1972 Bell and Ainsworth report. *Child Development, 48*, 1200-1207.

LeVine, R. A., Dixon, S., LeVine, S., Richman, A., Leiderman, P. H., Keefer, C. H., & Brazelton, T. B. (1994). *Child care and culture: Lessons from Africa.* New York: Cambridge University Press.

McKenna, J. J., & McDade, T. W. (2005). Why babies should never sleep alone: A review of the co-sleeping controversy in relation to SIDS, bedsharing, and breastfeeding. *Paediatric Respiratory Reviews, 6*, 134-152.

Miller, P.M., & Commons, M.L. (2010). The benefits of attachment parenting for infants and children: A behavioral developmental view. *Behavioral Development Bulletin, 10,* 1-14.

Pluess, M., & Belsky, J. (2009) Differential susceptibility to rearing experience: The case of childcare. *Journal of Child Psychology & Psychiatry, 50*(4), 396-404.

Richman, A., Miller, P., & Solomon, M. (1988). The socialization of infants in suburban Boston. In R. LeVine, P. Miller, & M. M. West (Eds.), *Parental behavior in diverse societies. New directions in child development*, No. 40. San Francisco: Jossey-Bass.

Soltis, J. (2004). The signal functions of early infant crying. *Behavioral and Brain Sciences, 27*, 443-490.

St. James-Roberts, I. (2007) Helping parents to manage infant crying and sleeping: A review of the evidence and its implications for practice. *Child Abuse Review, 16*, 47-69.

Teti, D.M., Kim, B.-R., Mayer, G. & Countermine, M. (2010). Maternal emotional availability at bedtime predicts infant sleep quality, *Journal of Family Psychology, 24*(3), 307-315. doi: 10.1037/a0019306

5

The Ethics of Early Life Care: The Harms of Sleep Training

Darcia Narvaez

Some argue that forcing babies into independent sleeping is good for them, increasing health and well-being. They argue that making babies learn to settle themselves at night helps them establish self-regulatory skills and makes them stronger. These practices are supposed to put babies on a road toward healthy physical outcomes, ensuring good sleep patterns. They are supposed to lead to emotional well-being, by ensuring children's ability to control themselves and establish self-reliance. These beliefs suggest that their advocates know very little about human development. It is a dangerous state of affairs.

What Do Babies Need and What Happens When We Ignore Those Needs?

Every animal has a developmental niche to promote optimal development in offspring. The niche represents a match between the needs of the offspring with environmental supports (i.e., parenting).

In comparison to other animal neonates, humans are still fetuses for 9 to 18 months after birth. This means that for at least 9 months postnatally their care should be as supportive and non-stressful as the womb. Because full-term infants are born with only 25% of the brain developed and many systems (e.g., immunity) are not fully functional for years, their early developmental niche is particularly influential, and is now known to affect long-term health and well-being (Shonkoff, 2012).

What Is Humanity's Evolved Developmental Niche?

Social mammals evolved a particularly intensive parenting style more than 30 million years ago, and until recently, humans have altered this only slightly. The components of the human evolved developmental niche (EDN) for early life include naturalistic birth (no separation of mother and baby, no induced pain or trauma), breastfeeding on demand for two to five years, nearly constant touch, responsiveness to the cues of the child, extensive positive social support including multiple adult caregivers, and free play with multi-aged mates.

Each of these factors is known to influence physical, mental, and psychosocial health. When the EDN is not followed, we can expect outcomes to be species atypical, not only in terms of health and well-being, but moral character (Narvaez, Panksepp, Schore, & Gleason, 2013; Narvaez, Wang, Gleason, Cheng, Lefever, & Deng, 2013).

If we turn to sleep training, we can see that it violates several characteristics of the EDN: (a) the infant is separated from adult bodies, which causes dysregulation of multiple systems; (b) breastfeeding on demand is made more difficult, depriving the child of the frequent bath of its hormones and body-building ingredients; (c) adults are, or are encouraged, to be too far away to be responsive, leading to distress and unanswered cues; and (d) the baby does not receive the social support it needs that builds a sense of self-confidence and trust. All told, the child's stress response, along with other systems, will be misdeveloped with long-term biopsychosocial-health effects.

Ethical Responsibilities

What Are the Ethical Obligations of Health Care Providers to Babies?

The field of medicine has several ethical principles to which its practitioners typically subscribe. These include respect for a patient's autonomy, beneficence (acting in the best interest of a patient), promoting justice, and non-maleficence (do no harm) (Beauchamp & Childress, 2001). Let's take these four principles and apply them to infant care.

Autonomy

Children have little capacity for autonomy as infants. However, their autonomy as adults can be undermined if early care is not responsive to their needs. How is that possible? With undercare, they are less likely to develop secure attachment, with its accompanying neurobiology for sociality. They are less likely to be self-controlled and intelligent, at least in social and stressful situations (Narvaez, forthcoming; Narvaez, Gleason, Brooks, Wang, Lefever, Cheng, & Centers for the Prevention of Child Neglect, 2013).

Beneficence

Beneficence means that healthcare providers should be acting in the best interests of babies. To do this requires familiarity with the EDN and the effects of not following it (Narvaez, Panskepp et al., 2013). Violations of this principle occur when medical professionals do not follow the EDN. Advocating separation of caregiver and baby, sleep in isolation, crying it out, are all practices that violate the principle of beneficence.

Justice

Justice and fairness for whom? Doctors seem ready to put adults' needs first, minimizing needs of babies. The understanding of infant development and the EDN may improve attitudes toward providing for the baby's needs. The rights of babies need to be placed centrally in the eyes of healthcare providers and parents.

Non-Maleficence

From the viewpoint of the EDN, the principle of non-maleficence is being continually violated by current medical practices and directives. One assumes that these violations are due primarily to misinformation (i.e., a lack of knowledge of the EDN). But recent publications seem to intentionally mislead parents about what is good for babies.

Recently, the AAP's journal published a poorly wrought paper that claimed: "Behavioral sleep techniques have no marked long-lasting effects (positive or negative)" (Price et al., 2012). The authors drew this very strong conclusion even though they looked at only one and not all possible effects. Moreover, they did not examine what the control group families were doing, even though there are decades of studies on mammals showing the long-term harm that distressing young offspring can have on mammalian brains.

We know from animal studies, and from properly conducted human studies, that cry-it-out techniques harm babies. Even when sleep training is used, and the baby stops crying for help, this does not mean the baby is not stressed (though a parent may feel fine because the baby is not crying). Cortisol levels in the baby are still high, doing their damage to young neurons (Middlemiss et al., 2012).

1. **What does extensive distress do to a baby?** It can kill neurons, and misdevelop brain systems that undergird self-regulation, self-concept, and emotional intelligence. When children are under-cared for, that is, when they do not receive what they evolved to expect (i.e., the EDN), they are more likely to develop increased stress reactivity from poorly developed vagal tone (Porges, 2011), HPA axis (Lupien et al., 2009), and misdeveloped gene expression (Meaney, 2001, 2010).

2. **What does isolating infants do to them?** It causes multiple systems to become dysregu-

lated, slowing down growth. Infants cannot self-calm, and so distress wreaks havoc on their development.

3. **What does encouraging parents to ignore signals from their infants do to the relationship?** It undermines parental sensitivity, one of the key factors for optimal child development in every domain studied.

4. **What are the long-term effects of sleep training?** We do not know. Studies never examine all factors, and some are sloppy in determining what they are assessing in the control and experimental groups (see Middlemiss et al., in prep). But there are numerous animal studies with other mammals showing that even short-term separation from the mother can have long-term detrimental effects.

The great ignorance and disdain for babies shown by both the authors of the aforementioned study, and the editors of *Pediatrics,* is alarming. By allowing this irresponsible and unethical conclusion, the editors are encouraging parents to do great harm to their children and our fellow citizens. Such actions demonstrate deep cracks in professional ethical responsibilities.

How Can Health Care Professionals Treat Babies Ethically?

The prism of ethics can be viewed in at least three ways: (a) following universal duties that anyone can carry out (i.e., the principles mentioned above), such as "do no harm"; (b) maximizing outcomes for all; and (c) taking virtuous action. We apply these approaches to the ethics of how adults (medical professionals and parents) might help babies sleep.

Do No Harm

The respect of persons often involves the principle of doing no harm (non-maleficence). Certainly we can agree that adults should try not to harm children. But then they require good information about what babies need. Babies need constant close contact with adults in early life. This suggests that health care providers ought to provide parents with alternatives to sleep training: ones that don't isolate babies from adult presence and touch.

Choose Actions that Result in the Best Outcomes for All Involved

A utilitarian approach attempts to maximize good outcomes for the greatest number of people. Certainly we need to be concerned for the needs of parents and supporting their well-being—exhausted parents are less able to take care of their children. However, babies have rights too. If you understand the EDN, you can see what rights babies should have, and how those rights are being violated routinely, even when there is no greater purpose for it.

Babies have the right to compassionate care from a welcoming community. They should not be subjected to painful experiences, such as cry-it-out techniques. They should not be isolated, untouched, or separated from the caregiver. Of course, they should receive the elixir of optimal development: breast milk. There are many other birthrights they should have too (see Narvaez , Panskepp et al., 2013).

Take Virtuous Action

Virtue involves behaving in the right way at the right time for the right reasons. Health care providers build their characters choice by choice. To be a virtuous professional means taking into account the whole context and one's impact in light of the type of profes- sional one wants to be. The character of a community is also built choice by choice, action by action. To be a virtuous community means taking the welfare of all into account and lubricating everyone's path to virtue. For babies' sleep, this means helping parents find ways that work without creating difficulties for themselves or their babies.

Ethical Problem Solving

What are the best sleep solutions for all concerned? The most important aspect to work on may be to circumvent sleep problems in the first place.

Decrease Precursors to Sleep Problems

Of course, not having a sleep problem in the first place would be the best approach. Thus, a prevention focus may do the most good. This means we need to look at the precursors to why babies won't settle down and take care of those. What do we know about unsettled babies? We know that not meeting a baby's needs is very distressing—needs for touch, presence, and calming by parents.

There are other factors that lead to sleep disturbances, such as infant irritability and maternal distraction. Addressing these issues can head off potential sleep problems in infants.

- Decrease stress on mothers during pregnancy (supporting moms with paid leaves from work and other support) (Davis et al., 2007).

- Decrease stress on babies at birth by figuring out alternatives to practices that harm them and their ability to cope (e.g., some childbirth drugs undermine settling).

- Establish on-demand breastfeeding immediately after birth.

- Help parents learn to enjoy keeping their babies close and carrying them with movement.

- Establish home routines for parents and babies early on that help babies sleep at night, such as exposure to light early in the day, and avoidance of light in the evening.

- Provide regular home visits for new parents with nurse practitioners and lactation consultants to ensure responsive parenting is established.

All these practices require community support. The whole society must step in to support babies and their families.

Treat Babies with Equal Respect

I have sometimes wondered whether healthcare providers have forgotten about the welfare of babies beyond keeping them alive. Remember, that not too long ago women were treated like children by medical professionals (and still sometimes are). African Americans were treated as inferiors. It is time for health care providers to change their attitudes and treatment of babies.

They should:

1. Treat babies as equal human beings who cannot yet express themselves in words.

2. Respect the evolved developmental niche and preserve it.

3. Find ways that respect babies first, then parents.

Challenging Myths and Changing Culture

Why is it that there is such a strong focus and belief on the notion that early care should foster self-reliance and independence? And how did people come to believe that such early care leads to healthy children and strong societies? Why, when all these assumptions are completely wrong?

It's not just that healthcare providers have lost sight of what babies need; American culture has shifted away from providing the kinds of support babies need. Since at least the 19th century, mothers have been advised by experts to not "spoil" their children with too much attention. The mostly male experts argued that "coddling" children would make them weak and whiny, so it was best not to touch babies and children too much. A U.S. government pamphlet urged mothers not to be inconvenienced by babies, letting them sit silently in their beds (Ladd-Taylor, 1986). Interestingly, baby experts in Germany in the early 20th century (during the rise of the Nazis) advocated the same types of cold-heartedness toward babies (Chamberlain, 1997; Dill, 1999).

Sleep "experts" also emphasized parental detachment from the baby. Parents were to be in charge, not the baby. We can see where these practices have brought us. In the last 50 years, not only has EDN childrearing continued to decline, but child well-being in the USA has become among the worst in the developed world, with self-regulation, mental, and physical health continuing to deteriorate. Those under age 50 have a health disadvantage compared to those in 16 other developed countries (Institute of Medicine, 2013). The U.S. has epidemics of mental health problems in all ages in the country.

Humans are the most complex organism, with the most extensive maturational schedule. What happens early often lasts a lifetime (Shonkoff et al., 2012). Because of this all adults have an ethical responsibility to facilitate children's optimal development. The professionals with first contact of baby and mother may be the most important to lead the way to a cultural change of *putting babies first.*

References

Beauchamp, T. L., & Childress, J. F. (2001). *Principles of bio medical ethics*. New York: Oxford University Press.

Chamberlain, S. (1997). *Adolf Hitler, die deutsche Mutter und ihr erstes Kind. Über zwei NS-Erziehungsbücher. Giessen, Germany: Psychosozial-Verlag.* ISBN 3-930096-58-7.

Davis, E.P., Glynn, L.M., Dunkel-Schetter, C., Hobel, C., Chicz-DeMet, A., & Sandman, D.A. (2007). Prenatal exposure to maternal depression and cortisol influences infant temperament. *Journal of the American Academy of Child and Adolescent Psychiatry, 46*(6), 737-746.

Dill, G. (1999). *Nationalsozialistische Säuglingspflege.* Einefrühe Erziehung zum Massenmenschen. Stuttgart, Germany: Enke Verlag. ISBN 3 43230711 X.

Institute of Medicine. (2013). *U.S. health in international perspective: Shorter lives, poorer health.* Retrieved from: http://www.iom.edu/~/media/Files/Report%20Files/2013/US-Health-International-Perspective/USHealth_Intl_PerspectiveRB.pdf

Ladd-Taylor, M. (1986). *Raising a baby the government way: Mothers' letters to the Children's Bureau 1915-1932*, New Brunswick, NJ: Rutgers University Press.

Lupien, S.J., McEwen, B.S., Gunnar, M.R., & Heim, C. (2009). Effects of stress throughout the lifespan on the brain, behaviour and cognition, *Nature Reviews Neuroscience, 10*(6), 434-445.

Meaney, M.J. (2001). Maternal care, gene expression, and the transmission of individual differences in stress reactivity across generations. *Annual Review of Neuroscience, 24,* 1161-1192.

Meaney, M. (2010). Epigenetics and the biological definition of gene x environment interactions. *Child Development, 81*(1), 41-79.

Middlemiss, W., Granger, D.A., Goldberg, W.A., & Nathans, L. (2012). Asynchrony of mother–infant hypothalamic–pituitary–adrenal axis activity following extinction of infant crying responses induced during the transition to sleep. *Early Human Development, 88*(4), 227-232.

Narvaez, D. (forthcoming). *The neurobiology and development of human morality.* New York: W.W. Norton.

Narvaez, D., Gleason, T., Brooks, J. Wang, L., Lefever, J., Cheng, A., & Centers for the Prevention of Child Neglect (2013). *Longitudinal effects of ancestral parenting practices on early childhood outcomes.* Manuscript under review.

Narvaez, D., Panksepp, J., Schore, A., & Gleason, T. (Eds.) (2013). *Evolution, early experience and human development: From research to practice and policy.* New York: Oxford University Press.

Narvaez, D., Wang, L., Gleason, T., Cheng, A., Lefever, J., & Deng, L. (2013). The Evolved Developmental Niche and sociomoral outcomes in Chinese three-year-olds. *European Journal of Developmental Psychology.*

Porges, S. W. (2011). *The polyvagal theory: Neurophysiologial foundations of emotions, attachment, communication, and self-regulation.* New York: W.W. Norton.

Price, A.M.H., Wake, M., Ukoumunne, O.C., & Hiscock, H. (2012). Five-year follow-up of harms and benefits of behavioral infant sleep intervention: Randomized trial. *Pediatrics, 130*(4), 643 -651. doi: 10.1542/peds.2011-3467

Shonkoff, J.P., Garner, A.S., The Committee on Psychosocial Childhood, Adoption, and Dependent Care and Section on Developmental and Behavioral Pediatrics, Dobbins, M.I., Earls, M.F., McGuinn, L., … & Wood, D.L. (2012). The lifelong effects of early childhood adversity and toxic stress. Pediatrics, 129, e232 (originally published online December 26, 2011).

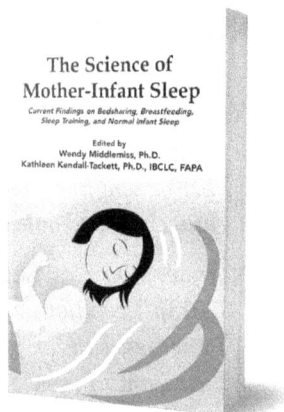

www.ingramcontent.com/pod-product-compliance
Lightning Source LLC
Chambersburg PA
CBHW060636280326
41933CB00012B/2056